Foreword

Hello my name is Anita I am 48 years old and married to my wonderful husband, Colin. We have two beautiful children, Grant age 27 and Kylie age 24. My son Grant is married to our lovely daughter-in-law Sammi, age 27 and they have two gorgeous children, Oliver age 4 years and Isabelle age 20 months. This book was written after I discovered that I had ovarian cancer. My grandson, granddaughter and I are very close and live in close proximity. They visit several times a week and were very aware that something was not right. This caused them enormous anxiety and if we addressed the issues with them initially, they were not able to take it on board. I am very lucky in the fact that I have worked with children and families for over 30 years and have good knowledge of their needs and understanding. I went onto the Macmillan website for tips on how to tell them, as this was too close for comfort, the more I tried to explain the worse it got. The information was invaluable and helped enormously. I borrowed a children's book from Macmillan called Mummy's lump, I adapted it so that it was relevant to my situation. The book was great as the story and pictures really helped. It was like watching the weight lift of Oliver's shoulders. Since reading the book we were able to prepare him for the treatment that I am undergoing, he is now able to talk openly about what is happening. Grandparents play an important role in children's lives and the impact that cancer has on families is very distressing, I hope that this book helps families support their young children in managing this stress as best as they can.

I researched books online and the staff at the Macmillan Centre at UCLH also searched for several weeks, to no avail. Young children need to be able to make sense of their world, reading them a story, opens the door for you and the children to have a discussion about what is happening. My grandson is 4 years old he was struggling with me losing my hair and when I decided to have it shaved off he helped shave it. We talked about what colour it would be when it grew back, he wanted blue hair. I set about finding a blue hair dye, unsuccessfully. When my hair started to grow back it was pure white, it had been brown before it fell out, (mostly out of a bottle you'll understand), he decided it was blue anyway, so it didn't really matter that I hadn't dyed it blue because he was content with it as it was. My point to this book is that whilst this is a difficult time for you and your family, it is important that the children are helped to understand why mummy, daddy, siblings, nanny, grandad, aunts and uncles are stressed, because understandably they will be and children will pick up on it, however young they are. This book is dedicated to my grandchildren Oliver age 4 and Isabelle age 20 months. I would like to say a massive thank you to my wonderful husband, daughter, son, daughter-in-law, family, friends, Macmillan and all the staff of UCLH. You are all amazing and your help has been invaluable. Thank you for keeping me strong.

前言

你好！我的名字是Anita，48歲，與體貼的丈夫Colin育有一對秀麗的兒女，27歲的Grant和24歲的Kylie。Grant 與可愛的27歲妻子Sammi，有兩名漂亮的孩子，4歲的Oliver和20個月大的 Isabelle。這本書寫於我患卵巢癌之後。孫子和孫女住在附近，與我關係非常緊密。他們每週來我家幾次，非常警覺任何事情不對勁。若我們一開始跟他倆談我的病，他們不會明白而且會很焦慮。我十分慶幸自己有超過30年的兒童及家庭工作經驗，瞭解他們的需要和認知能力，但由於彼此關係緊密，我越解釋反而弄巧反拙。我瀏覽Macmillan網站，找到十分寶貴和大有幫助的資料。我借了一本兒童書名叫《媽媽的腫塊》，略略改編故事內容以適切我的情況，並配合書中圖畫向他倆講述後，我感覺Oliver如釋重負。自從一起閱讀此書，我們幫助他準備好面對我將接受的治療，現在他能公開講述所發生的事。癌症對家庭的震撼令人非常愁苦，而祖父母在兒童的生命裏扮演了重要的角色。我期望此書能幫助眾家庭支持他們年幼的子女，以最佳的方法去處理這壓力。

兒童能感受身邊成人的焦慮，程度上不會低於你希望保護他們免患癌症，保護他們免受癌症帶給家庭的震撼。你避免在他們面前或向他們談及癌症，事實上卻引來他們對未知事情的焦慮。我期望此書能幫助你，猶如它幫助我的孫兒一樣。

當我的頭髮脫掉時，我的4歲孫子感到困擾。我決定剃掉頭髮，並讓他與他的媽媽幫我剃髮。我們談到頭髮再長出來會是甚麼顏色，他希望是藍色。我四出尋找藍色染髮劑卻找不着。以前我的頭髮是染了棕色，當頭髮重新長出來卻是純白。無論如何，他認為是藍色，但我有沒有染藍色都不要緊，只要他像從前一樣感到滿足就是了。我想藉此書說明的是，幫助兒童明白，為何媽媽、爸爸、嫲嫲、爺爺、姨姨、叔叔感到壓力，是十分重要的。因為無論他們是如何年幼，亦會明白和感受到周遭所發生的事。

此書獻給我的 4 歲孫兒 Oliver 和 20 個月大的 Isabelle。 我衷心感謝我體貼的丈夫、女兒、兒子、媳婦、家人、朋友、Macmillan和所有 UCLH 的職員。你們非常了不起，對我的幫助是無價寶。多謝你們 幫助我繼續堅強。

嫲嫲有癌

My Nanny has cancer

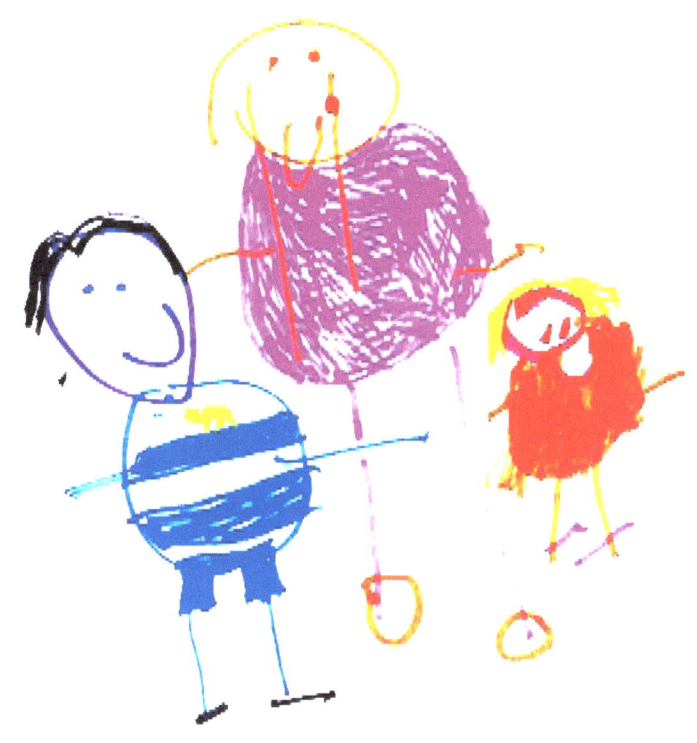

Written by Anita Hudson

嫲嫲有癌症

Illustrated by Oliver Hudson

Oliver and Isabelle live with their mummy and daddy and their dog called Ziggy

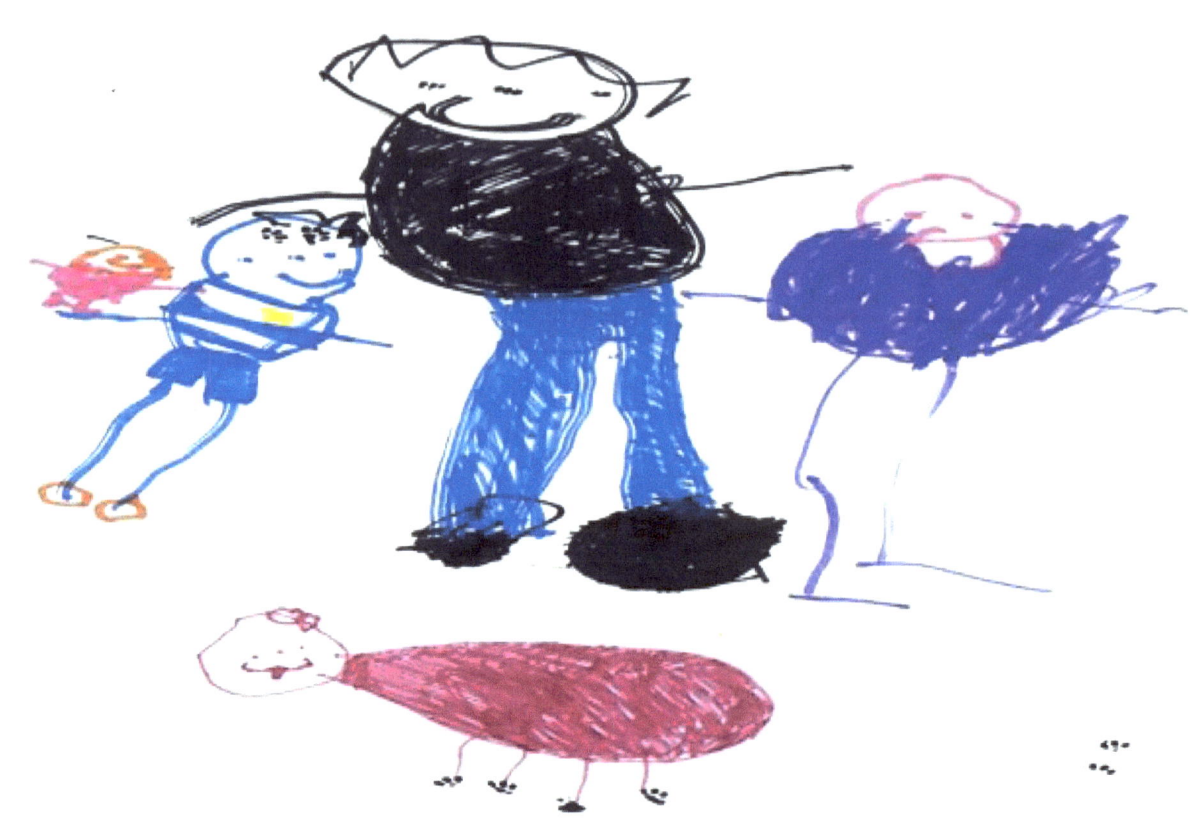

爸爸、媽媽、妹妹和我住在一起，還有狗狗Ziggy。

Nanny and grandad live close by and we visit them a lot. Sometimes they look after us. Isabelle and I love visiting them.

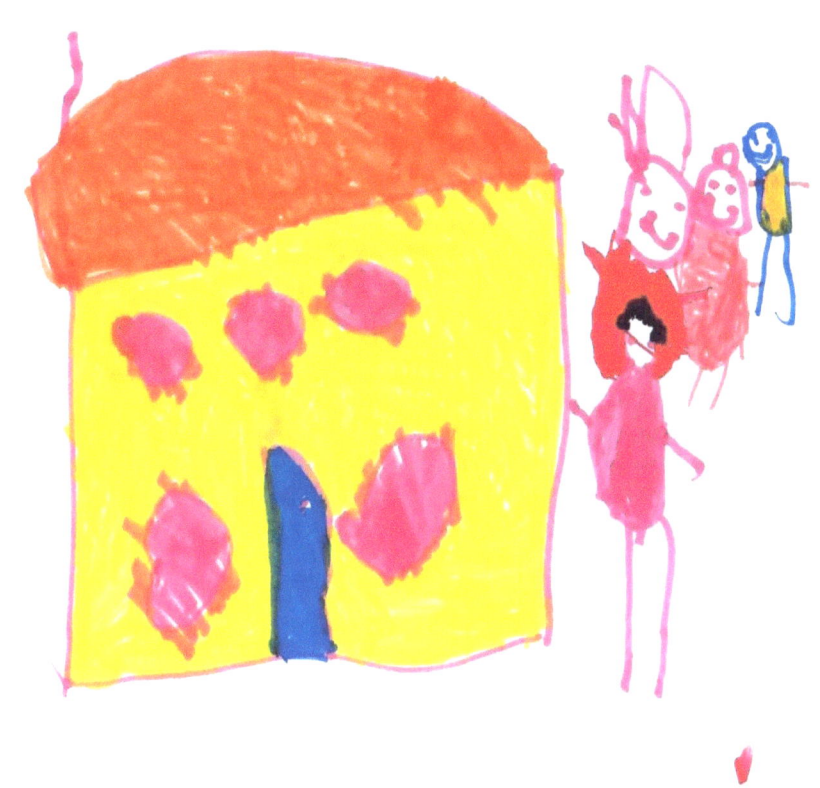

爺爺和嫲嫲住在附近，我們經常探望他們。
有時他們照顧我倆。我和妹妹喜歡探望他們。

Nanny has a treat box in the cupboard, we get to choose something every time we visit.

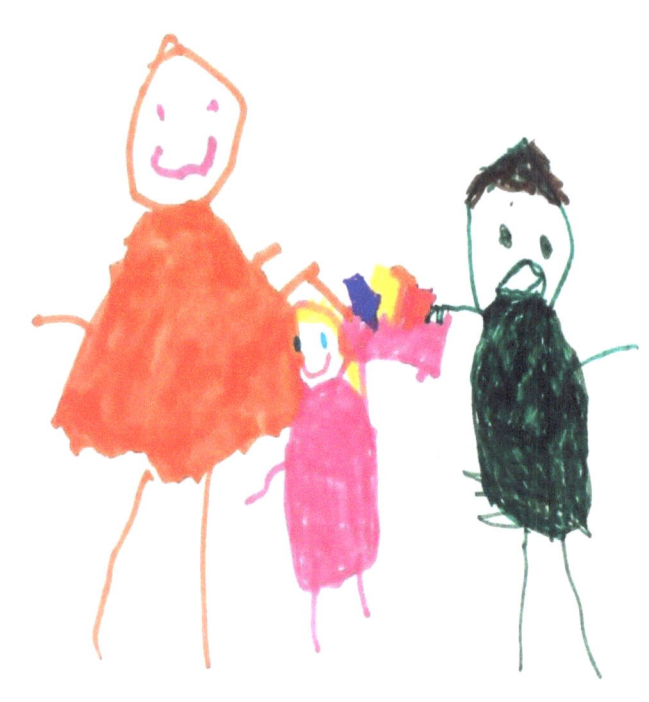

嘛嘛的杯櫃裡有個零食盒，每次探爺爺嘛嘛，
我們都可以選取一些來吃。

那裏還有個玩具箱，我倆喜歡倒空它。妹妹常常爬進去。

There is also a toy box which we love to empty out. Isabelle always climbs in.

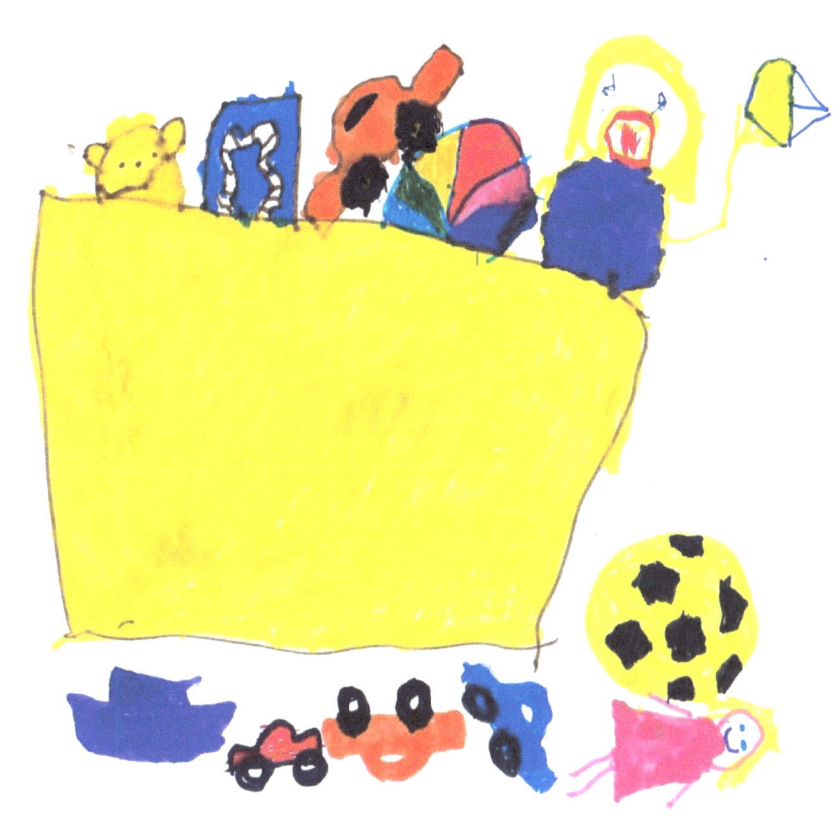

What is your favourite thing about visiting nanny and grandad?

當你探望爺爺嫲嫲，最喜歡的是甚麼？

某天，嫲嫲肚痛要看醫生。醫生說嫲嫲生了腫塊叫癌症。

One day nanny had a tummy ache. She went to the doctor.

The doctor said that nanny has bad lumps called cancer.

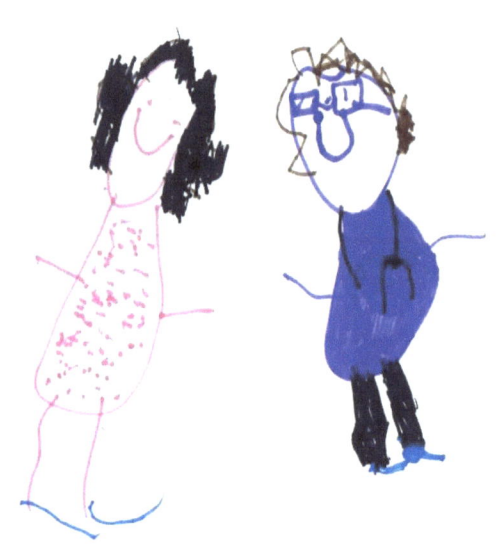

我們會感染傷風或水痘，但不會感染癌症。無人知道為甚麼有癌症。這不是任何人的錯，並非我們頑皮或對人不好便會有癌症。有時我也會肚痛，但跟嫲嫲的不相同。

You can't catch cancer like a cold. No one knows why it happens. It isn't anybody's fault. Cancer doesn't happen because you have been naughty or cross with someone, it just happens. Sometimes I get tummy ache but it is not like nanny's.

Nanny feels sad, grandad, auntie, mummy and daddy are worried.

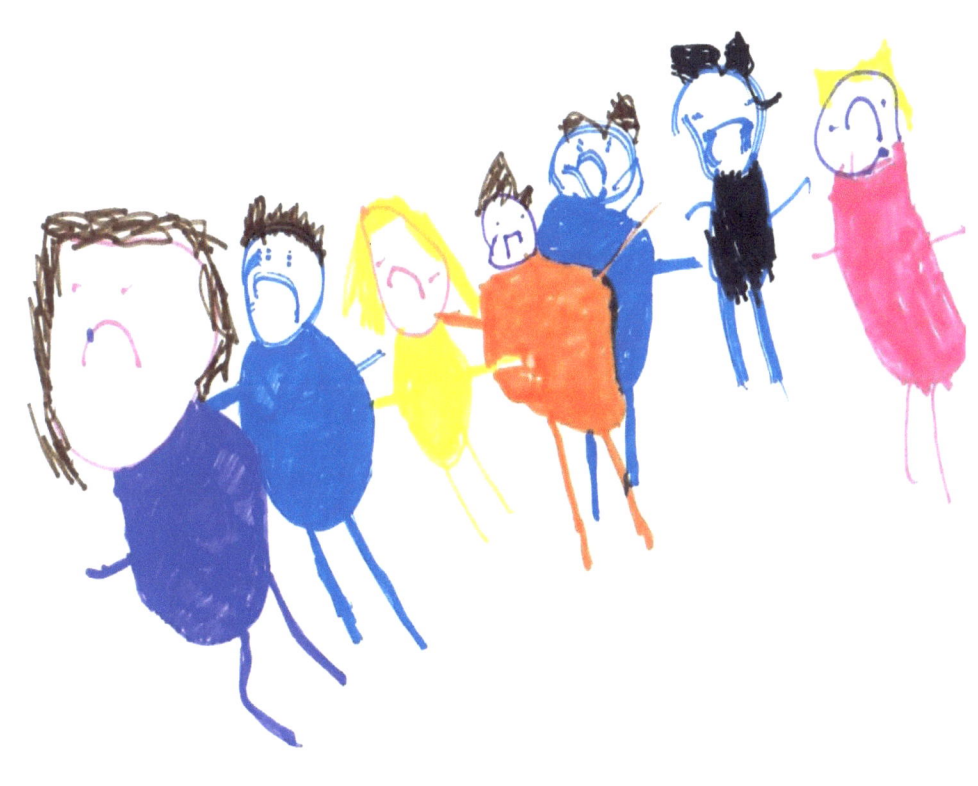

嫲嫲難過，爺爺、阿姨、爸爸和媽媽都擔心。

醫生說嫲嫲一定要到醫院做手術，取走那塊叫腫瘤的腫塊；否則腫塊變得更大，令嫲嫲十分辛苦。

The doctor says nanny must go to the hospital to have an operation and take the bad lumps, called tumours away. Otherwise they will grow bigger and make nanny very poorly.

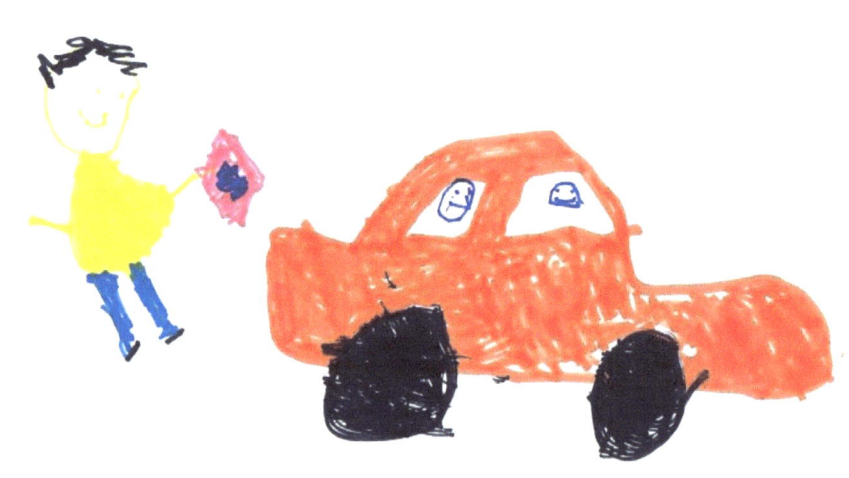

Grandad takes nanny to hospital for a few days. I don't like it when nanny isn't at home, it makes me feel sad. I know that nanny has to go to the hospital to get better though.

爺爺帶嫲嫲去醫院住幾天。我不喜歡嫲嫲不在家，感到難過。

不過，我知道嫲嫲必須去醫院才能好轉。

我畫了兩幅圖畫給嫲嫲放在醫院牆壁。

嫲嫲喜歡我的圖畫，令她微笑。

I gave nanny two pictures that I drew for her to put on the wall at the hospital. Nanny loves pictures they make her smile.

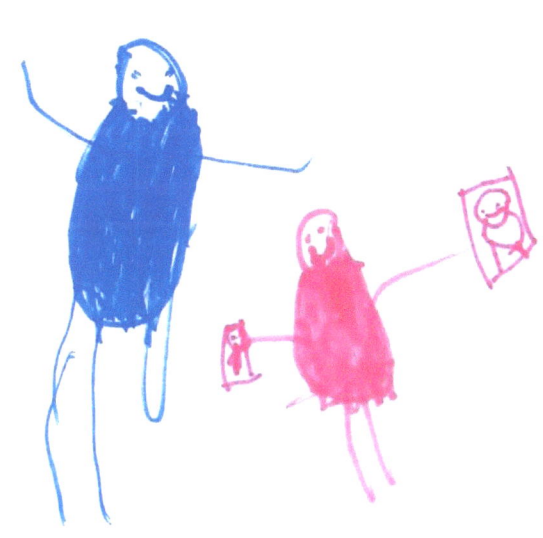

甚麼會令你的嫲嫲微笑？

What makes your nanny smile?

When nanny has her operation she is given an anesthetic so it doesn't hurt when they take the tumours away. The nurses look after nanny.

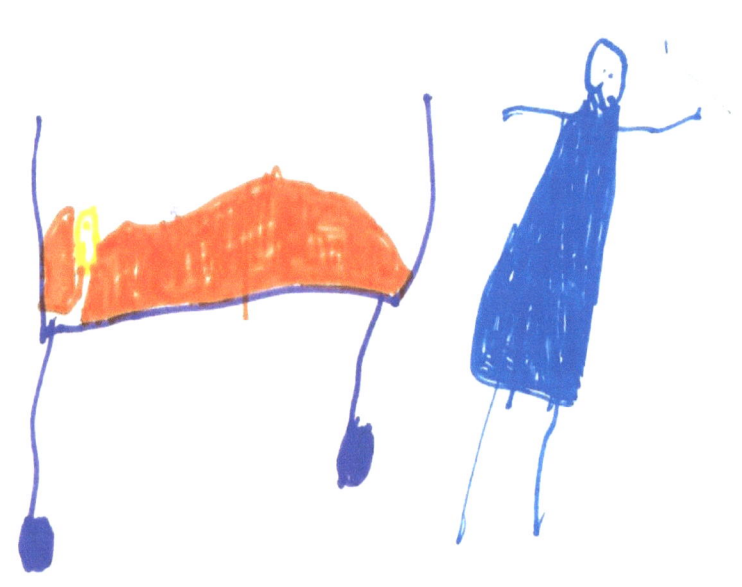

嫲嫲做手術切掉腫瘤時，麻醉藥會令她不感到痛楚。護士會照顧嫲嫲。

當嫲嫲感覺好一點，爸爸媽媽帶我和妹妹到醫院探望她。嫲嫲喜歡我畫的圖畫，放在她旁邊的牆上。我的圖畫令嫲嫲感到好一點。

When nanny is feeling a bit better, mummy and daddy take me and Isabelle to the hospital to visit her. Nanny loves the pictures that I drew for her and has them on the wall next to her. They make nanny feel better.

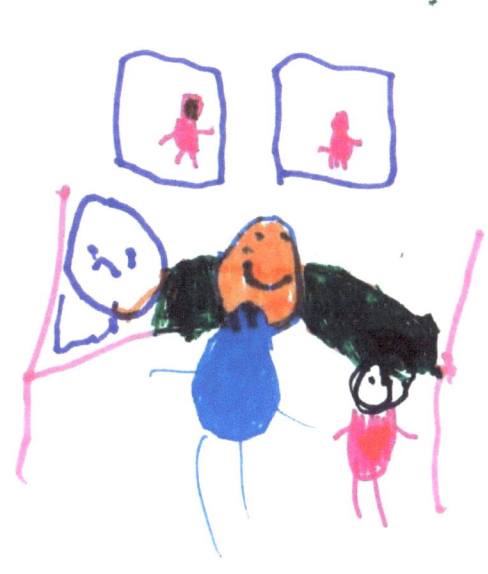

探望嫲嫲時，請問您會做甚麼令嫲嫲開心？

What would you like to do to cheer nanny up when we visit?

爺爺做所有家務和煑晚飯。他觸動了煙霧探測器，
令我大笑起來。我說：「啊，爺爺！」

Grandad is doing all the jobs at home and cooking dinner. It makes me laugh when grandad sets off the smoke detector, I say "oh grandad".

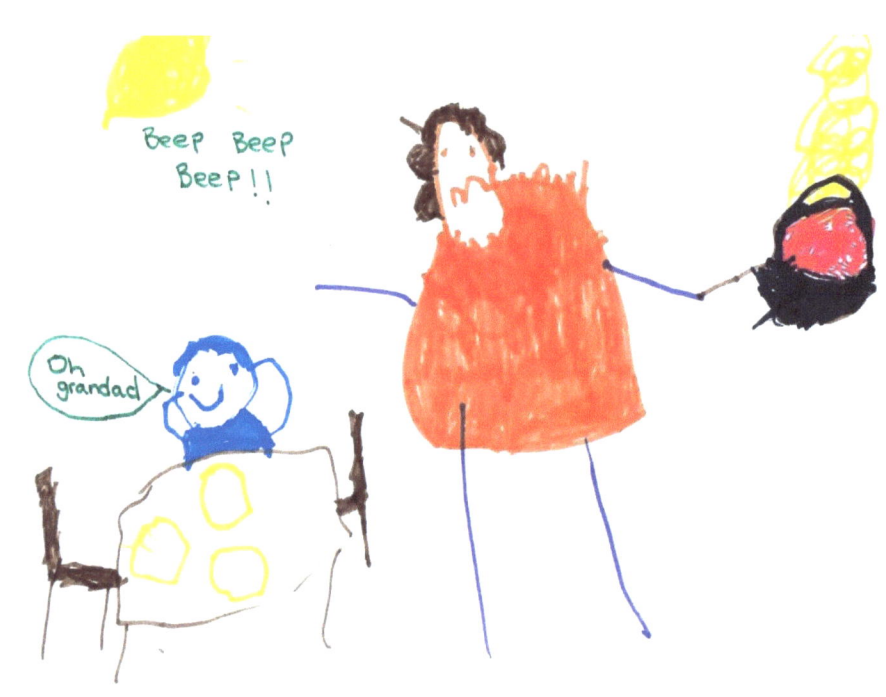

爺爺做甚麼會令你笑？

What does your grandad do that makes you laugh?

When nanny comes home she needs lots of rest, her tummy is sore where the professor cut the cancer out.
I am careful with nanny and give her my gentlest kisses and my biggest squeezes go to grandad.
When nanny is not sore anymore, I will share my biggest squeezes between her and grandad.

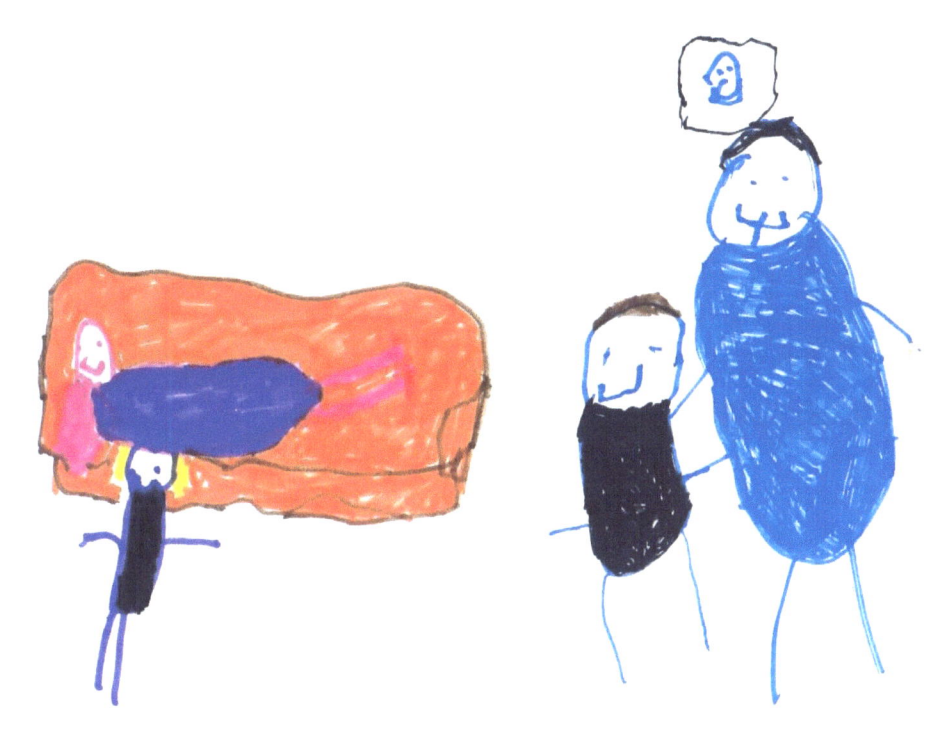

當嫲嫲回家，她需要多休息。教授在她肚子酸痛的地方切掉腫瘤。我小心和溫柔地吻嫲嫲，用最大力擁抱爺爺。如果嫲嫲不痛了，我會跟嫲嫲和爺爺分享我的最大力擁抱。

我跟爺爺玩遊戲。當嫲嫲好一點，她就會同我玩遊戲。

妹妹和我喜歡與嫲嫲和爺爺玩遊戲。

I play games with grandad and when nanny is better she will be able to play games with me again. Isabelle and I love to play games with nanny and grandad.

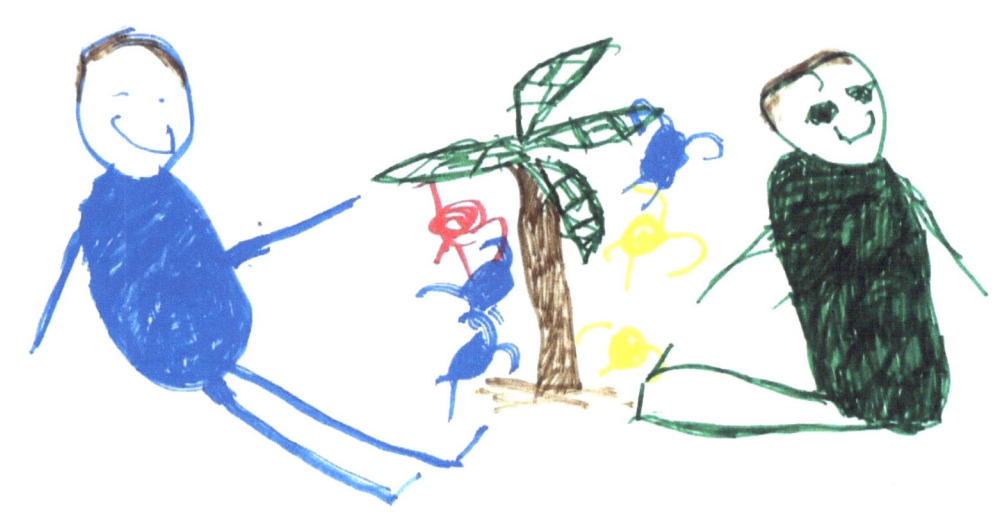

你最喜歡與嫲嫲和爺爺做甚麼？

What do you like doing best with nanny and grandad?

嫲嫲需要一些強效藥物名叫化療，阻止腫塊再生長，不像你家裡的藥，乃是護士在醫院給她的特別藥。這些藥令她感到噁心和困倦，不想多玩。有時化療令嫲嫲感到很沮喪。妹妹和我給她擁抱，令她感覺好一點，因為嫲嫲仍然喜歡擁抱。

Nanny has to have some strong medicine called chemotherapy to stop the lump growing back. It's not like medicine that you have at home it is special medicine that the nurses give to her at the hospital. It makes her feel sick and tired, and she doesn't want to play much.

Sometimes it makes her feel down in the dumps. Isabelle and I give her cuddles to help her feel better, cos she still likes cuddles.

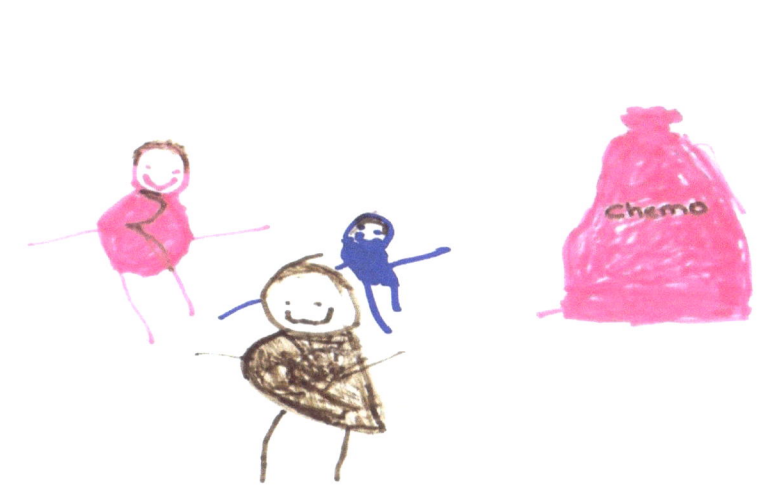

What could we do to help nanny feel better?

我們可以做甚麼幫助嫲嫲感到舒服？

Chemotherapy makes nanny's hair fall out. Nanny wears pretty hats. My friend's nanny likes to wear wigs. Nanny's hair will grow back when she stops having the chemotherapy.

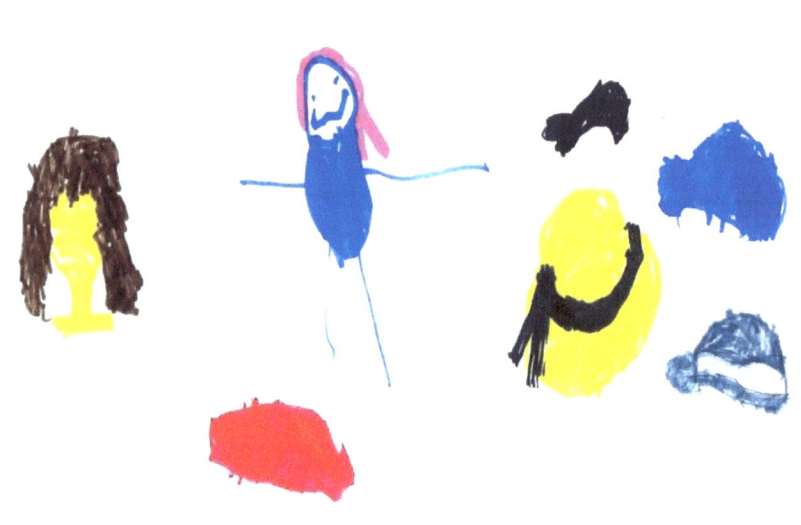

化療令嫲嫲頭髮掉光了，她戴著漂亮的帽子。我朋友的嫲嫲喜歡戴假髮。當停止化療，嫲嫲的頭髮會重新長出來。

嫲嫲說，重新長出來的頭髮可能會顏色不同或捲曲。

我希望嫲嫲的頭髮長成藍色，這是我最喜歡的顏色。

Nanny says it might grow back a different colour or curly. I hope nanny's hair grows back blue, it's my favourite colour.

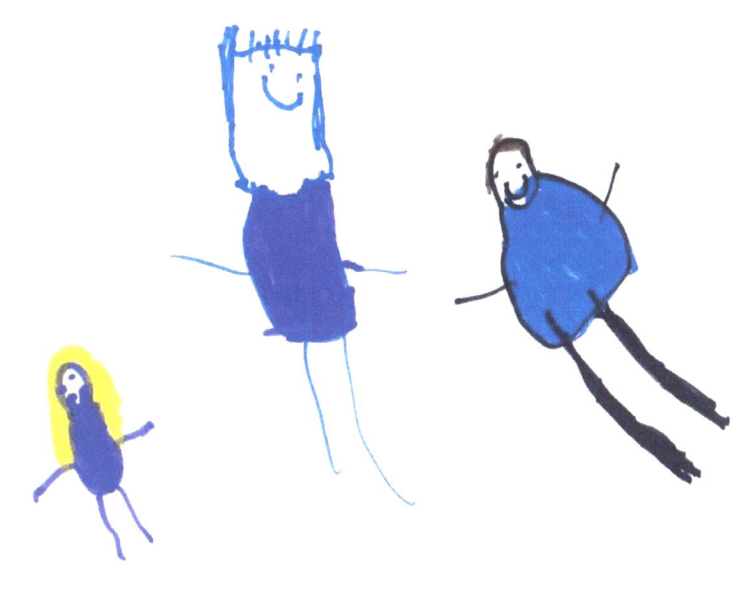

你認為嫲嫲重新長出來的頭髮會是甚麼顏色呢？

你最喜歡甚麼顏色？

What colour do you think nanny's hair will grow back?

What is your favourite colour?

The doctor will see nanny often to check that the bad lumps haven't come back.

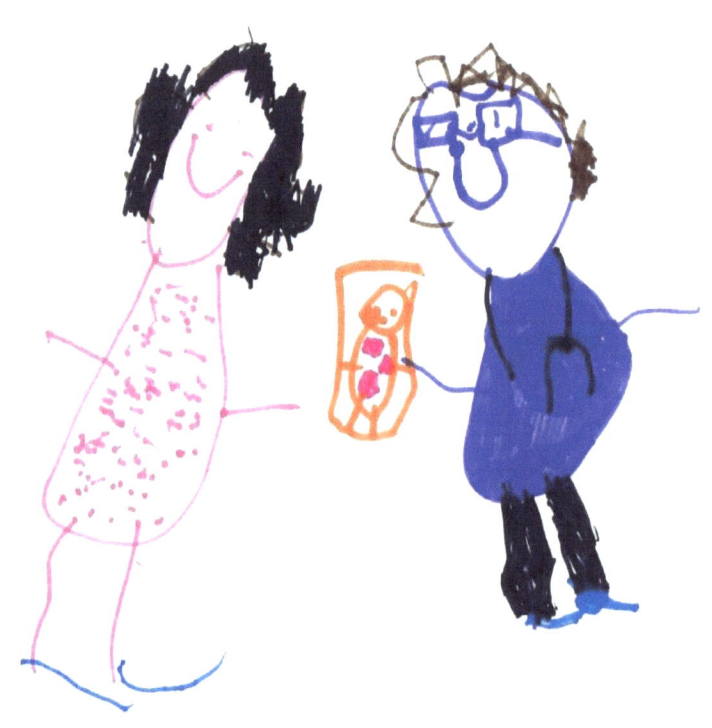

醫生會經常為嫲嫲檢查，看看那些壞腫塊有沒有再長出來。

最後，嫲嫲的治療結束了，我們都感到開心。嫲嫲和爺爺帶我們去公園。我騎自行車，妹妹坐上她的嬰兒車去。我們玩鞦韆、攀爬架和滑梯，非常快樂。

At last nanny's treatment is finished and we all feel much happier. Nanny and grandad take us to the park. I ride my bicycle and Isabelle goes in her buggy. We have fun on the swings, climbing frame and slides.

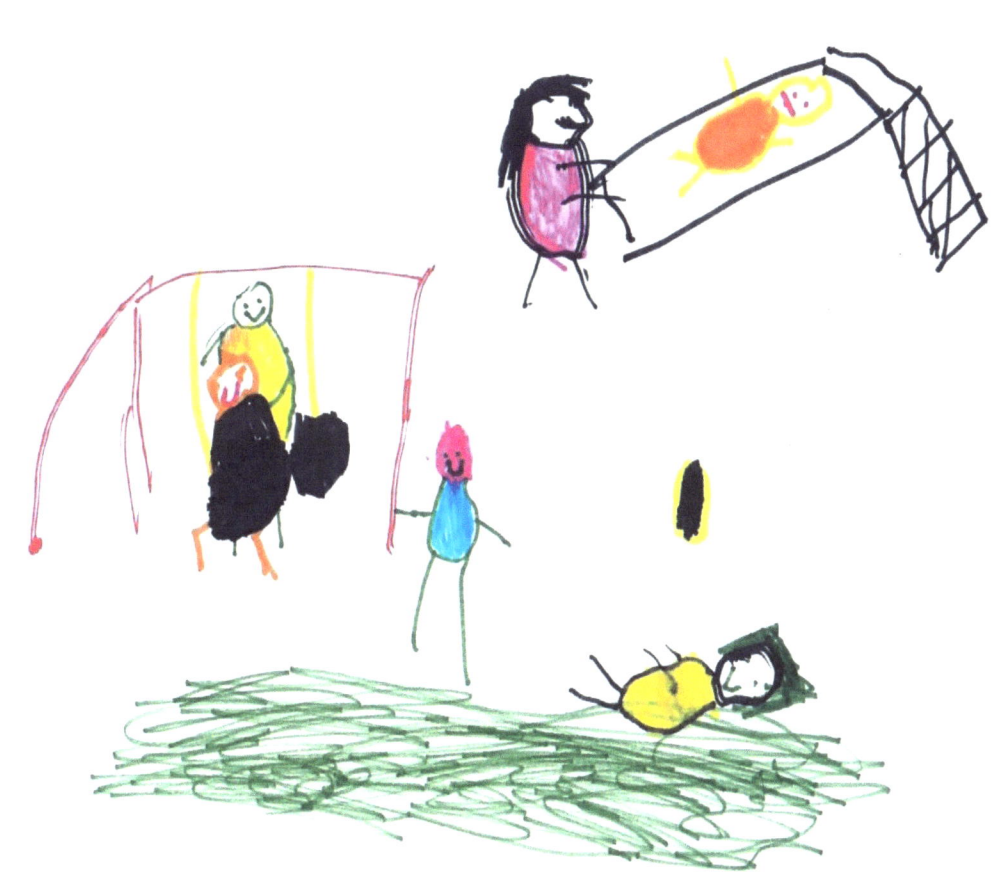

你最喜歡在公園做甚麼？

What is your favourite thing to do at the park.

Here are some examples of how to explain cancer to young children (taken from the Macmillan website, explaining cancer to children): 'I have a lump growing inside my body (explain which part) that shouldn't be there. It's called cancer and I'm going to have an operation to take it away. After that, the doctor will give me medicine so that the lump doesn't come back.'

下面是如何向幼童解釋癌症的例子: **(**取自麥美倫網站，向兒童解釋癌症**)**

「我的身體長了一塊不應該存在的腫塊（説明身體那部分），

叫做癌症。我要做手術把它拿走，然後醫生會給我開藥，令這 腫塊不再長出來。」

Tips for parents and grandparents: Give your child as much information as they need using simple words in a way that they understand. Remember to change nanny to whatever it is that they call you or their grandparent, grandma, Nanna etc.

給父母和祖父母的提示：

儘量給你的孩子有關資訊，要用他們能理解的簡單詞語。

記得將「嫲嫲」改換成他們以往對患癌親人的稱呼：例如 公公婆婆、爺爺嫲嫲、爸爸媽媽等。

Children pick up on stress so be aware that it is natural for them to react to it. You may notice a change in their behaviour. It is important that whilst being sensitive to their needs they will continue to need clear boundaries and routines, this helps them feel secure. I know it is very tempting to give in to their demands and want to over protect them, however this will lead to insecurities for them and a whole load of extra stress for you.

孩子們會感受到壓力，所以要留意，他們的反應是很自然的。

您可能注意到他們的行為有所改變化。敏銳他們需求的同時，

讓他們清楚知道自己的界限和生活常規是重要的，這令他們有

安全感。身為家長有很大的試探，就是對孩子的要求讓步和過

份保護他們，然而這將會增加他們的不安全感和你的壓力負荷。

* 'I have an illness called cancer. The doctor is giving me medicine to help me get better. The medicine might make me feel sick or tired some days, but other days I'll feel fine.' 「我有一個叫做癌症的疾病。醫生開藥幫助我康復。這種藥可能令我有幾天感到不舒服或疲倦，但其他日子我會感覺很好。」

* If your child asks you what cancer is - 'our bodies are made up of lots of tiny things, called cells. They all have a different job to make our bodies work and keep us healthy. Cancer is when some cells stop working properly and stop the healthy cells doing their jobs. The cancer cells can grow into a lump.'

如果你的孩子問你甚麼是癌症-「我們的身體是由許多微小的細胞

組成，各自有不同的工作，讓我們的身體運作和保持健康。癌症就是當一些細胞停止正常工作和阻止健康細胞正常運作。癌細胞能長 成腫塊。」

Important points to get across: Children often worry about things like causing the cancer or catching it. All children need reassurance that: * Nothing they did or thought caused the cancer * Cancer isn't like a cold you can't catch it - it's ok to sit close, hug or kiss * There will always be someone to take care of them * They can always ask questions and talk to you about how they feel * You'll listen to their worries and try to help them cope. 傳達的要點：

孩子們常常擔心自己感染或引致癌症之類的事情。 所有的孩子都需要得到保證： *
並非他們所做或所想引致癌症 * 癌症不像感冒，你不會感染到癌症 -
靠近坐、擁抱或接吻都無問題 * 一定有人照顧他們 *
他們可以隨時提出問題，與你談談他們的感受 * 你會傾聽他們的憂慮，並設法幫助他們應付。

My grandson is 4 years old, I informed him of the cancer in simple terms, listening to his questions and answering them as simply as possible. I found the Macmillan website invaluable when discussing the cancer with him. He was able to understand what was happening and talk openly about it.

孫兒四歲，我用簡單詞句將癌症告訴他，聆聽他的問題，並
儘可能簡單地回答。與他討論癌症的時候，我發現麥美倫網
站非常有幫助。他能明白發生了甚麼事，並開放地談論。

The book was a god send, because it was able to support what I had told him and he could understand what was happening to me. I wish you the very best with your treatment. Stay strong and remember to keep the children informed in a way they will understand. Written by Anita Hudson

這本書是一份禮物，幫助我告訴他究竟我發生了甚麼事，讓他能理解明白。
我祝福你獲得最好的治療。
保持堅強，記得要隨時用孩子們能理解的方式，告訴他們發 生了甚麼事。 **Anita Hudson** 著

www.ingramcontent.com/pod-product-compliance
Lightning Source LLC
Chambersburg PA
CBHW041311180526
45172CB00003B/1064